Thinking Outside the Diet Box: A Revolutionary New Way to Approach Weight Loss

Henry Solomon

Published by Henry Solomon, 2023.

THINKING OUTSIDE THE DIET BOX: A REVOLUTIONARY NEW WAY TO APPROACH WEIGHT LOSS

First edition. April 17, 2023.

Copyright © 2023 Henry Solomon.

ISBN: 979-8223185949

Written by Henry Solomon.

Introduction
The Importance of Rejecting the Diet Mindset

Have you ever looked in the mirror and saw something you didn't like? We all have.

"Dieting" has become a way of life for so many that it is no surprise that weight loss is a multi-billion-dollar industry always throwing out the newest, latest and greatest diet scheme to take off the excess pounds.

The diet mindset is a way of thinking that encourages people to focus on their physical appearance and weight, rather than their overall health. It promotes the idea that dieting and restricting food intake are the only ways to achieve a healthy lifestyle. Unfortunately, this mentality can have serious consequences on an individual's health and well-being. Rejecting the diet mindset is essential for promoting healthy eating habits and developing a positive relationship with food.

There are numerous plans and fad diets out there that promise fast and easy results. However, these weight loss plans and fad diets are both harmful and useless for our weight loss agenda. The truth is that these plans and diets are often ineffective and can even be damaging to our health, so, how do we lose the weight *AND* keep it off?

We must change our mindset completely and change our lifestyle. Instead of "dieting" for the sake of losing, we should change our lifestyle for the sake of gaining.

For starters, these types of diets can be very restrictive, severely limiting the types of food we can eat and the number of calories we can consume. This can lead to nutrient deficiencies, as well as feelings of deprivation and frustration. Additionally, these diets are often based on a one-size-fits-all approach, which can be inadequate for an individual's metabolic needs.

Furthermore, these diets may seem to work for a little while, only to bring the weight back and more than when we started. This is due to the fact that these diets are not sustainable in the long-term, and our body may also go into "starvation mode", where it attempts to store calories and fat as it believes it is being deprived of food.

The only way to ensure lasting weight loss is to make changes to your lifestyle that you can maintain in the long-term. This includes eating a balanced diet that incorporates all food groups, as well as getting regular physical activity. Additionally, it is important to address any underlying emotional or mental health issues that may be contributing to your weight gain.

It is time to take back our lives and our minds that are held captive by dieting and instead, enjoy a lifestyle change that will make all the difference where we can finally enjoy all the benefits that permanent weight loss brings to the body, mind, and spirit.

If you feel like your diet is taking over your life and controlling what you eat, it is time to break free from diet culture. Breaking free from diet culture can be a difficult process, but it doesn't have to be.

Diet culture has become pervasive in our society, but it doesn't have to control us! Taking the necessary steps to break free from diet culture can help us reclaim our lives and our health. Here are five steps you can take to break free from diet culture:

1. Unfollow and Unfriend: Social media can be a major source of comparison and body shaming. Take a look at who you are following and what you are consuming on social media, and unfollow or unfriend anyone who perpetuates diet culture or body shaming.
2. Ditch the Diet: If you are on a diet, it's time to get off of it. Diets don't work; they can actually be detrimental to your health. Instead, focus on making healthier choices that make you feel your best.

3. Get Educated: Learn more about Intuitive Eating and Health at Every Size. These concepts can help you make peace with food and your body.
4. Celebrate Your Body: Take the time to appreciate and celebrate your body. Do things that make you feel good and make your body feel loved.
5. Speak Up: Speak up when you hear someone promoting diet culture or body shaming. It can be uncomfortable, but it's an important step in breaking free from diet culture.

By taking these five steps, you can start to break free from diet culture and reclaim your life and health.

Struggling to Lose Weight?

The weight loss struggle describes how people struggle with healthy permanent weight loss. One of the main elements that adds to this struggle is the mass amounts of crash and fad diets that promise fast weight loss.

Within the context of trying to stay healthy, losing weight has proven to be an incredibly difficult challenge for many people, especially when it comes to keeping the weight off permanently. The truth is that the amount of weight lost is not the only determining factor of success; the key is in maintaining the weight loss over a long period of time.

Weight loss is a common goal that many individuals strive to reach. Unfortunately, it can be a difficult journey to travel. Obesity is a growing epidemic in the United States and many individuals struggle to break free from the cycle of overeating and inactivity. Weight loss is a battle that requires dedication, perseverance, and the right tools.

There are numerous plans and fad diets out there that promise fast and easy results. However, these weight loss plans and fad diets are both harmful and useless for your weight loss agenda. The truth is that these plans and diets are often ineffective and can even be damaging to your health, so, how do you lose weight *AND* keep it off?

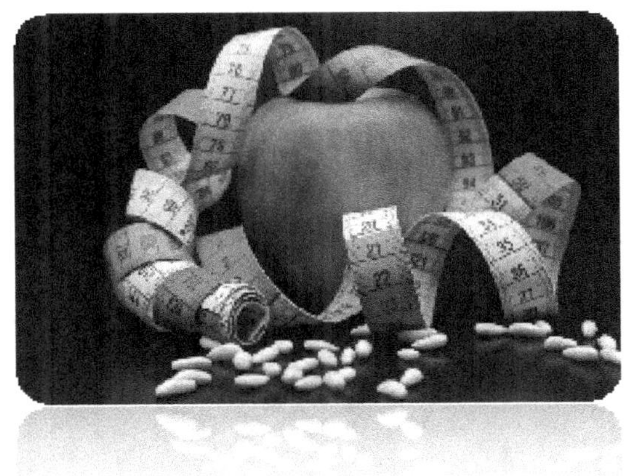

Researchers hypothesize that the consumption of processed food, increasing stress levels, and unhealthy lifestyle choices play a key role in the large numbers of individuals being overweight.

Eating a variety of healthy foods that are high in fiber and protein and low in sugar and fat can help to reduce cravings and keep you feeling full longer.

If your ultimate goal is to lose weight to be healthier and maintain a healthy weight, then a short-term fix is not for you. Instead, you need to learn and practice weight management, which is never accomplished with some amount of dedication and will power.

Weight loss is a journey that requires dedication and perseverance. With the right tools, it is possible to break free from the cycle of obesity, maintain a healthy weight level, and ultimately, lead a healthier lifestyle.

There are a number of reasons why you may be struggling to lose weight, and understanding these factors can help you work to make changes that will help you reach your goals.

While it may be hard to stay on track, there are some strategies that can help you keep the weight off permanently.

First and foremost, it is important to have realistic goals and expectations. If a person sets unrealistic goals and expectations, they are more likely to give up if they don't reach them. A healthy weight loss goal should be to lose 1-2 pounds per week. This is a realistic goal and allows for individuals to adjust their lifestyle and eating habits while slowly make progress.

Another important strategy to keep the weight off permanently is to create a balanced diet. Eating a balanced diet that includes all food groups is essential for weight loss and maintenance.

Here are some of the reasons you may be feeling the weight loss struggle.

- **Poor Diet**
  Too often, people focus on cutting calories without properly evaluating the nutritional value of what they are eating. Eating too much of the wrong foods, such as processed or fast food, will make it harder to lose weight. Eating a balanced diet of whole foods that include lean proteins, healthy fats, and complex carbohydrates is essential for weight loss.
- **Lack of Exercise**
  Exercise is an important part of any weight loss plan, but many people don't get enough. Aim to include both cardio and strength training to maximize the benefits.

- **Stress**
  Stress can be a major factor in weight loss resistance. When you are feeling overwhelmed, it can be difficult to make healthy choices. Make sure to prioritize self-care and relaxation to help manage stress and make it easier to reach your goals.
- **Not Enough Sleep**

Sleep is an important part of your overall health and weight loss plan. Getting enough quality sleep can help keep your hormones regulated and your energy levels up, which can make it easier to make healthy choices and stick to your plan.

- **Unrealistic Expectations**
  Setting unrealistic expectations can lead to disappointment and make it hard to stay motivated. Don't expect to lose weight quickly; focus on gradual progress and making realistic lifestyle changes that you can stick to in the long-term.
- **The Temporary Mindset**
  One of the reasons that the typical "diets" fail is that they are temporary conditions, hence phrases like "I am getting on a diet," or "I just got off a diet." Permanent weight loss is the opposite, it is not a temporary state, and so it cannot be achieved with temporary solutions.

- **The "I'm starving!" Binge**

After your crash diet ends, you all of a sudden find yourself starving. Your body is out of whack and your stomach is screaming at you. A cheat day can't hurt, right? So you binge. This cycle becomes a habitual process that you can't seem to escape.

- **You are not Balanced**

You may find yourself avoiding some food altogether as your crash diet says, thinking it will aid you in the process. However, this is not the case. Your body needs all food groups in their own right to stay healthy and therefore manage your weight.

- **Lack of Knowledge**

Many simply do not understand what it means to live a healthy lifestyle, which includes, what to eat, and how to expend calories.

Making changes to your diet and lifestyle can be difficult, but understanding the reasons you may be struggling can help you make the necessary adjustments. With commitment, dedication, and a little bit of patience, you can reach your weight loss goals.

Ditch The Diet Mindset

As if you need more convincing. Have you been trying to lose weight for years and still have not been successful? If so, it might be time to ditch the diet mindset and start looking at weight loss from a different perspective.

Fad diets can seem like a quick fix, but they rarely work in the long run. Instead of following strict rules and restrictions, focus on making small, sustainable changes that will help you reach your goals without feeling deprived or overwhelmed.

By understanding how your body works and what it needs to stay healthy, you can create an individualized plan that fits your lifestyle and helps you lose weight for good.

Here are some reasons why you need to ditch the diet mindset and start living!

Better For Your Health

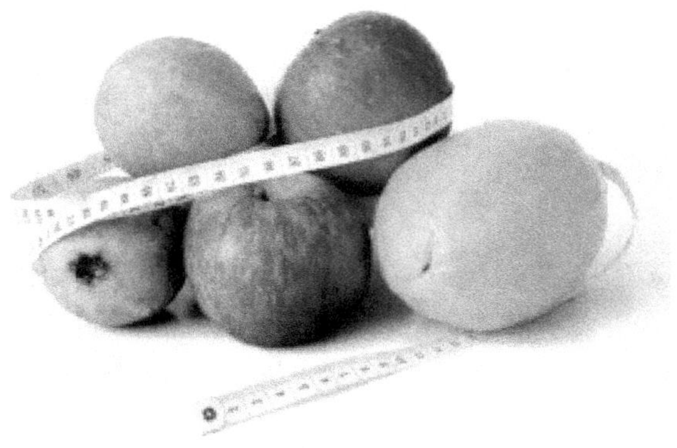

The diets don't work. Plain and simple. Instead, they offer you the shiny proposal of fast weight loss, as long as you do not eat anything but eggs, or drink anything but wine. However, a lifestyle change gives you the tools needed to lose weight naturally and slowly, without giving anything up. Your health will improve as you begin to eat healthier foods and lose weight. You will save yourself the headache, frustrations, and larger health risks associated with fad diets and yo-yo dieting.

Better For You

Your health is very important. However, just as important as your health is your wellbeing. Your thoughts, your feelings, and your complete emotional health are also important and can be compromised.

By changing your lifestyle, you can affect your emotional health positively instead of negatively.

Losing weight and maintaining a healthy weight is likely to improve your life in numerous ways.

A study of participants in the National Weight Control Registry (https://www.nwcr.ws) found that subjects who were able to achieve and maintain significant weight loss improved not only their physical health, but also mobility, energy levels and self-confidence.

If your self-confidence is wavering due to your weight or simply, the need to be healthier, you may need a lifestyle change. Weight management is better for you and your health.

You will benefit overall from ditching the temporary diet mindset and focusing on changing your eating habits for the long term. The National Weight Loss Registry noted that 98% of participants were successful in achieving their weight loss goals by modifying the food they consumed.

If you are ready to make this decision, know that you will not be disappointed. It will not happen overnight; it will be hard work, but you will feel better as soon as you commit to being persistent in achieving your weight loss goals.

Weight Loss and the Fad Diet - The Yo-Yo Dieting Horror Show

Have you ever felt like you have been on a never-ending journey of dieting while trying to achieve weight loss without any lasting results? If so, you're not alone. Many people struggle to lose weight and keep it off because they're stuck in the diet mindset.

The truth is, diets don't work. They often lead to yo-yo dieting, where you lose a few pounds only to gain them back shortly after. To break this cycle and achieve lasting weight loss, it is important to ditch the diet mentality and focus on making sustainable lifestyle changes that will help you reach your goals.

People often want to lose weight rapidly but there is a risk of malnutrition, or of giving up and putting on more weight than before.

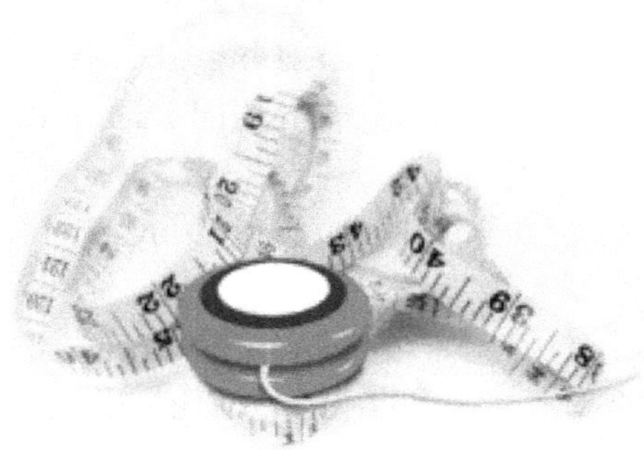

How many times have you said or thought...

"Next week I start my new diet"

"My new year's resolution (like last year and the year before) is to start a new diet"

"I need to get back on my diet"

"I need to find a new diet that really works"

"I'm going to stuff myself this week because next week I start my new diet."

Yo-yo dieting or weight cycling is defined as small spurts of weight loss as a result of some diet, and then a regain of the weight, and then another diet and more loss and regain, which develops into a vicious and never ending cycle.

For example, you are able to lose five pounds quickly by quitting carbohydrates altogether. However, the next week, you binge and gain the five pounds back plus an extra two. You start the process over again and this time, you gain even more. This type of dieting is damaging to your health.

Studies have shown weight cycling (yo-yo dieting) to have certain health risks, including the likelihood of developing high cholesterol, high blood pressure and gallbladder disease. They also state that this type of dieting can have a negative effect on your psychological health as well. You soon fall under the spell that what you are doing is healthy for you, although it is not.

The small successes feel good only to be met with larger gains that make you feel bad. Eventually, you may decide that your lifestyle with any diet is better than this horrid cycle, but that is far from the truth.

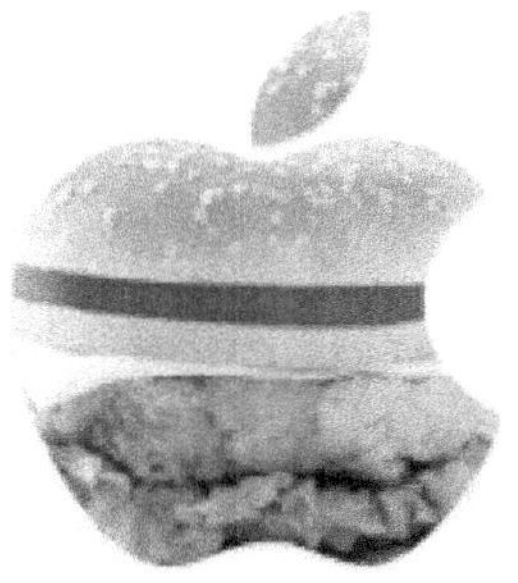

There are serious diseases associated with being obese:

- High blood pressure
- Heart disease
- Stroke
- Type 2 diabetes
- Certain types of cancer
- Arthritis
- Metabolic syndrome
- Complications and risks for premature death from belly fat
- Gallbladder disease
- And others

Yo-yo dieting also includes risks to your health, including:

Increased Risk Factors for Disease

The extreme calorie restriction commonly seen in yo-yo dieting increases cortisol, a stress hormone that causes negative effects on the body over prolonged periods of its existence including, increasing risks for developing type 2 diabetes, cancer and heart disease.

Weight Gain

While yo-yo dieting may deliver results in the short term, over the long term most will regain the weight. Researchers at UCLA have found that dieting is not only ineffective, but can often make you gain more weight than you originally had after a small loss of usually only 5 to 10%.

Less Muscle, More Fat

Extreme diets that restrict mass calories lead to loss of critical lean muscle mass, and once the diet is over, the dieter is left with less muscle and more fat.

Less Energy

Yo-yo dieting is believed to actually slow metabolism, which results in low energy levels and hinders the body's natural ability to burn calories throughout the day. When the body is deprived of the calories it needs to function, it makes adjustments that can result in fatigue, irritability and limited brain function.

You try one diet only to find yourself gaining the weight back. So, you try another. That one doesn't work either. This cycle repeats over and over until you are in the middle of a yo-yo lifestyle.

This is why it is important to change your lifestyle instead and get off the yo-yo diet merry go round.

10 Reasons Why Fad Diets Do Not Work

Fad diets are a dangerous trend that promises quick weight loss and improved health outcomes. Unfortunately, these diets are often unsustainable and have not been scientifically proven to be effective.

Fad diets usually involve extreme changes in eating habits, such as drastically reducing calories or eliminating entire food groups. Although these diets may lead to short-term weight loss, they are not sustainable in the long run, and the weight that is lost is often regained as soon as the dieter returns to their normal eating habit.

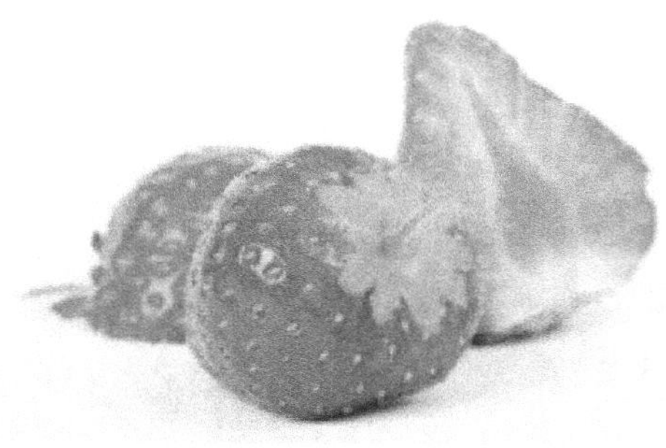

Fad diets are often marketed as a quick fix for weight loss, but in reality, they don't work. Here are 10 reasons why fad diets don't work:

1. Fad diets are often restrictive, eliminating whole food groups or certain types of foods. This can lead to nutritional deficiencies and an unbalanced diet.
2. Many fad diets are based on eating one type of food or a combination of foods that are not good for you, such as processed foods or foods high in sugar.
3. Fad diets are often unsustainable and not realistic in the long term. People who follow these diets often gain the weight back

once they stop the diet.

4. Fad diets can be expensive and sometimes require people to buy special ingredients or supplements.
5. Fad diets usually don't provide enough calories or the right balance of nutrients for healthy weight loss.
6. Fad diets can make you feel deprived, which can lead to binging and overeating.
7. Fad diets can be dangerous for people with certain health conditions, such as diabetes, kidney disease, and heart disease.
8. Fad diets can cause dehydration and electrolyte imbalances due to lack of fluids and essential minerals.
9. Fad diets can lead to muscle loss due to lack of protein.
10. Fad diets can cause depression or anxiety due to the strict rules and restrictions they impose.

The Permanent Weight Loss Formula

It bears repeating here that permanent weight loss is a goal that many people try to achieve but often find hard to maintain. There is no one-size-fits-all formula for weight loss, but there are several key strategies that can help you stay on track for long-term success.

The key to successful, permanent weight loss is making small changes and creating healthy habits that will last for life. With a few simple strategies, you can achieve permanent weight loss and keep it off for good.

Now that you are aware of the negative side effects of crash dieting and the positive side effects of a lifestyle change, you are ready to ditch the diet mindset and begin a new lifestyle.

HOW ABOUT MAKING HABIT CHANGES AND NOT WEIGHT LOSS YOUR GOAL?

✓ Instead of focusing on the weight, you are focusing on your mindset
✓ Another temporary diet versus a new lifestyle
✓ Diets are temporary but lifestyle changes are permanent

How Empowering Is This?

In essence, this means that you will no longer be starting, and restarting and restarting a new diet. You will instead begin to make profound eating and lifestyle changes, even if you start small, like eliminating soda.

Now, keep in mind that when you make profound changes in your eating habits (more on these below) you will lose weight and keep it off. It is really that simple.

Most important you will NEVER have to diet again, you can just live!

By investing in a lifestyle change, you are making the decision for better health and an overall better life.

Getting Started

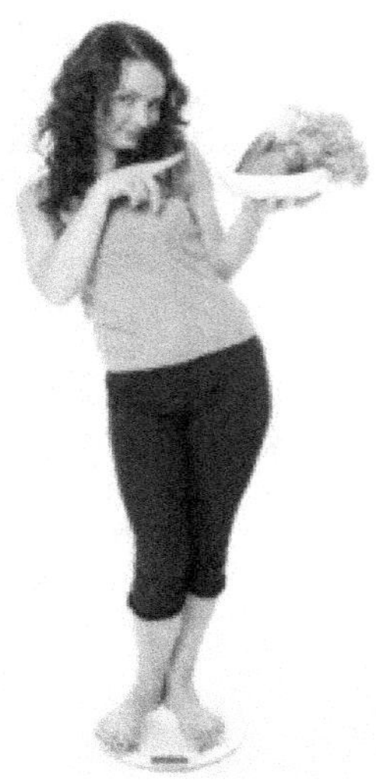

If you are ready to change your life, then there are important and useful facts you need to know that will assist you on this new path. These key aspects will aid you in losing weight gradually and keeping it off for good.

Calories In – Calories Out

The "calories in versus calories out" model is a popular way of looking at how to achieve and maintain a healthy weight. The basic idea behind this model is that if the number of calories you take in matches the number of calories you expend, your weight should remain stable. In other words, if you consume the same number of calories as you burn, your weight should stay the same.

This can include anything from fruits and vegetables to junk food and sugary drinks. It is important to note that not all calories are created equal, and different types of food can have different effects on your weight and overall health.

The "calories out" part of the equation is the number of calories you burn. This can be affected by your level of physical activity, as well as your basal metabolic rate, which is the number of calories your body uses just to stay alive. Exercise can be an important part of burning calories, but even things like standing and walking can help you burn calories.

To lose weight however, you need to burn more calories than you eat.

It is important to remember that the "calories in versus calories out" model is just one way of looking at weight management. Other factors such as diet quality, sleep, stress, and genetics can also play a role in your overall health and weight. Additionally, some people may find that the "calories in versus calories out" model doesn't work for them. If this is the case, it is important to talk to a healthcare professional to find a plan that works for you.

Overall, the "calories in versus calories out" model is a popular way of looking at how to achieve and maintain a healthy weight. By understanding the different components of this model, you can make sure that you are getting the right balance of calories and activity in order to reach your goals.

Simply put, the "calories in versus calories out" is a very simple formula that allows your body to make the adjustments it needs to lose weight naturally and more importantly, gradually.

The Centers for Disease Control state that evidence falls in favor of lower and more gradual weight loss in keeping the weight off.

This method of weight management focuses on healthy weight loss instead of fast weight loss.

The rule of thumb is to burn more calories than you eat, so whatever calories come in must also come out or be expended through the use of energy.

The formula:

1 pound = 3,500 calories

To lose 1 pound of week: reduce caloric intake by 500 calories per day; to lose 2 pounds a week: reduce caloric intake by 1000 calories per day.

- Take calories in through eating healthier
- Burn calories out through exercise and being active
- Create a deficit

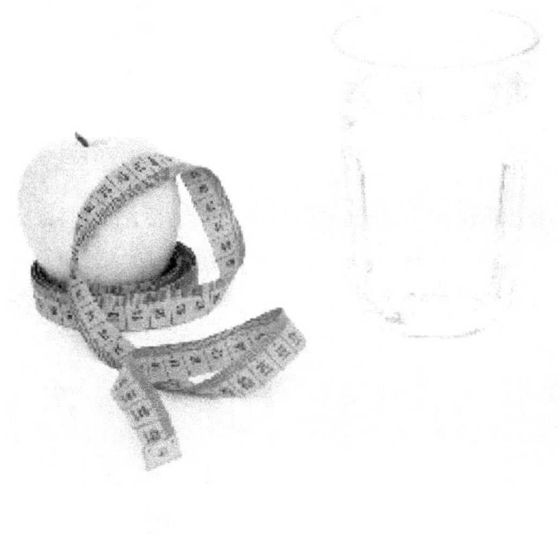

The amount of calories needed daily will vary from person to person and also depends on age, weight, and activity levels.

This means that someone who works out an hour every day will be able to eat more calories than someone who is sedentary.

There are plenty of online calculators to help you figure out your perfect number (https://www.calculator.net/calorie-calculator.html).

How Science Determines Calorie Count in Food

Calorie counting is a popular way to monitor what you eat and maintain a healthy diet. But it can be difficult to know exactly how much energy is in a particular food item. Fortunately, there is a scientifically proven method for determining the calorie count of any food.

The first step of the process is to weigh the food item you want to measure. This ensures that the amount of food is consistent and accurate for the experiment. It is also helpful to measure the food in grams for accuracy.

The next step is to combust the food item. This can be done using a calorimeter, which is a device that is designed to measure how much energy is released when a food is burned. The calorimeter captures the heat released and converts it into a calorie measurement.

The third step is to calculate the amount of energy released. This can be done by multiplying the weight of the food item by its specific heat capacity, which is an indication of how much energy it takes to heat up a certain material. The result is the total amount of energy released when the food is burned, which is its calorie count.

Finally, the calorie count can be converted into a more useful measurement. For instance, it can be converted into kilocalories (kcal), which is a unit of energy that is often used in nutrition labels.

By following this scientific method, anyone can accurately measure the calorie count of any food item. This can be a useful tool for those who want to monitor what they eat and stay healthy.

Calorie Count

- Protein: 4 kilocalories per gram
- Carbs: 4 kilocalories per gram
- Fats: 9 kilocalories per gram
- Alcohol: 7 kilocalories per gram

How The Body Uses Calories

The body uses calories as a source of energy to perform various functions, such as breathing, digestion, muscle movement, and other metabolic processes. When we consume food, the body breaks down carbohydrates, fats, and proteins to release energy in the form of calories.

These calories are then converted into ATP (adenosine triphosphate), which powers the body's cells. Any extra calories that are not immediately needed are stored as glycogen or fat for future use. The amount of calories needed by the body varies based on individual factors such as age, gender, height, weight, and activity level.

One of the issues with using the bomb calorimeter method is our bodies do not always use or "burn" every calorie it takes in.

Fiber is a good example, where the insoluble fiber is not fully digested, and so those calories aren't truly absorbed and you actually consume less than what you'd expect based on the count. By the way, this is a great reason to eat high fiber foods.

Not All Calories Are Equal

Calories are NOT created equal as the exact same amount of calories from two different types of food yield completely different biological effects in the body.

Are 182 calories worth of soda the same as 182 calories worth of kale?

- 182 calories in a 22 ounces portion of soda
- 44 grams of sugar
- And no other nutrients

Soda is a carbohydrate and once inside your body the sugar from the soda will be quickly absorbed causing a rush of sugar to your blood stream and a subsequent spike in blood glucose levels. Other adverse chemical reactions in the body will take place, including the storage of belly fat, and increases in bad cholesterol.

Since soda or any sugar is an insulin trigger, that flood of insulin blocks the appetite controlling hormone leptin, which registers satiation, and when leptin is blocked this leads to overeating, and out of control cravings for junk food leading to a never-ending cycle of unhealthy eating with cravings that are never truly satisfied.

Additionally, soda affects the appetite hormone ghrelin that sends a signal in the body when it has received food, and since soda is not registered as food, just the empty sugar calories, this leads to increased hunger, and no true satisfaction.

If that's not enough, any sugar that is not used for energy will be stored as fat. Notice that soda offers absolutely no nutritional value.

What About the Kale?

- 33 Calories per 1 cup; (182 calories = 5 cups)
- Potassium
- Protein
- Vitamin A
- Calcium
- Iron
- Fiber
- Vitamin C
- Vitamin B-6
- Magnesium
- Key antioxidants

Kale is also a carboxylate but unlike the soda, kale will digest slowly in the body, will not cause sugar spikes, and provides a wide array of nutrients helping to heal and energize the body and prevent chronic disease.

None of the calories form kale will turn to fat, even if you ate the whole 5 cups or even 10 cups, so unlike the soda it will never contribute to weight gain.

Kale's nutritional profile and fiber will satisfy hunger, and never cause out of control cravings for junk food.

Essential nutrients, like potassium, protein, iron, vitamin D, and magnesium, heal the body, unlike the soda that wreaks havoc and causes harm.

Keep in mind the above applies when comparing all other empty calorie foods, like cookies, and French fries to all non-starchy vegetables, proteins, and whole grains.

One study evaluated the correlation between sugar and calories to risks for type 2 diabetes, and concluded that the addition of an extra 150 calories a day hardly increased the risk for the disease, but when those calories came from soda the risk increased by 700%.

Healthy Eating

You may agree that eating healthier is the only way to go. However, what exactly does it mean to "eat healthy"? Obviously, portion control is crucial. However, it also means to eat clean. Clean eating means eating whole real food, such as vegetables, eggs, lean meats, fruits and whole grains.

Whole food is food that is unprocessed and eaten in its natural state, for example:

- ✓ An apple is a whole food, but apple pie is not
- ✓ A chicken breast is whole food, but chicken tenders are not
- ✓ Grilled cod is whole food, fish sticks are not

Whole food provides you essential nutrients to nutrify your body and eliminates any unnecessary additives and calories that make up processed food.

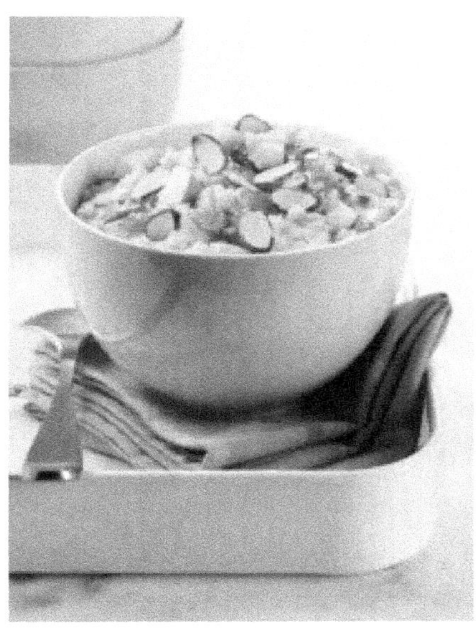

For a balanced eating plan to be successful, you need to:

- Eat plenty of vegetables
- Enjoy healthy fats, like avocados, nuts, and olive oil
- Eat whole grains in moderation
- Eat protein which includes lean meat, fish, poultry, eggs and soy alternatives
- Include low or nonfat dairy - milk, yogurt, cheese or alternatives
- Drink plenty of water
- Limit saturated fat and avoid all trans fats
- Limit your alcohol intake
- Reduce sugar as much as possible, this also means eating low sugar fruits like berries in moderation.
- Reduce processed food

Reasons To Choose Clean Whole Food

You may be thinking that if the formula for weight loss is calories in calories out, then what's the difference what you eat.

Real whole food such as fresh vegetables, lean protein, and whole grains are nutrient dense foods that provide your body with energy, support internal body process and allow you to eat clean.

Junk food and processed food is filled with empty calories that offer no such nutritional value. One of the key motivational aspects of reaching your goal weight and staying there is that you feel good, as well as look good. Eating clean ensures this, while eating junk food will only drag you down and interfere with healthy digestion.

To equal the same amount of calories as the 22-ounce soda, you would need to eat 5 cups of kale, and this applies to all vegetables and other junk foods, so think about how much more food you can actually eat when choosing quality food?

Your Best Choices

✓ Eat foods that are slow to digest, like high fiber vegetables, lean meats and eggs

✓ High fiber food supports weight loss and weight management. Plant foods are great sources of indigestible fiber that's calories don't count because that fiber is not absorbed in the body. Eat lots of vegetables, and low sugar high fiber fruits like berries

✓ Protein foods, such as fish, meat, chicken and turkey have no fiber so they will count more than vegetables and should be eaten in smaller portions

✓ Healthy fats, such as nuts, avocado and olive oil are necessary for optimal health, since they are high in calories, they should be moderated and eaten in the smallest portions as compared to protein and vegetables

✓ Eat real whole food, this means nothing boxed or made in a factory. Shop the periphery of the super market, in the produce, meat, and dairy aisles

✓ Moderate the simple sugars, such as junk food, cookies, cakes, and processed food and this also means eating fruit in moderation since it is high in sugar

As you can see, not all calories are created equal, and changing eating habits to reflect the above considerations will allow you to reach your weight loss goal and stay there.

Profound Changes in Eating Habits

It is important to understand that as you choose wisely your eating habits will change. These profound changes in your eating habits are most important to your new lifestyle.

A single patty cheeseburger contains roughly 303 calories. A veggie burger contains roughly 124 calories. That makes for a 179 calorie difference within your day. This is a profound change without giving your taste buds a break. If you eliminate the cheese from that burger, you will save about 80 calories.

If you drink soda every day, you can save a whopping 1,050 calories each week by simply cutting out **just one can** from your day.

If you substitute vegetables for potatoes or French fries in at least 1 meal per day, you will save more than 800 calories a week, and will begin to change your taste towards healthier choices.

Evaluate what you eat each day, write it down, and begin to choose healthier options. Start small if you must, but keep going until you reach your goal.

These types of profound but small changes will result in weight loss and a strengthening of your self-confidence and empower you to continue making smart decisions to keep you on your path.

Make smart choices, do your research, and fill your plate with real whole food.

Remember: you are making habit changes instead of weight loss your goal

Portion Control

Portion control and weight loss go hand-in-hand. Many people struggle with their weight because they simply eat too much. Portion control is the process of controlling the amount of food you consume each meal. It can be a powerful tool for weight loss, as it can help you to reduce your calorie intake and reach your goal weight.

When it comes to portion control, the most important thing is to pay attention to the size and quantity of food that you're eating. This can be accomplished by measuring out your portions before you eat or by using smaller plates. It is also important to be mindful of the food choices you make, as some foods are higher in calories than others. For example, instead of a large plate of French fries, opt for a smaller portion of vegetables, such as a side salad.

In addition to changing your portion sizes, it is important to be mindful of the timing of your meals. Eating smaller, more frequent meals throughout the day can help to keep your blood sugar levels balanced and reduce cravings. This can also help you to stay full throughout the day and avoid overeating.

It is important to remember that portion control isn't an all-or-nothing approach. You don't have to completely eliminate certain foods or completely avoid certain foods. Instead, focus on reducing the portion size of certain foods and eating a balanced diet. This can help you to reach your goal weight while still enjoying the foods you love.

Here are some tips to help you measure and control portion size:

1. **Use a food scale:** A food scale can be an invaluable tool when it comes to measuring and controlling portion sizes. It is important to weigh foods to get an accurate measurement of the amount you are consuming.

2. **Use smaller plates and bowls:** Using smaller plates and bowls can be an effective way to control portion sizes. By using

smaller plates and bowls, you can help prevent overeating and ensure you are consuming the appropriate amount of food.

3. **Read food labels:** Reading food labels is a great way to get an accurate measurement of portions. Food labels provide information about the amount of calories, fat, and other nutrients per serving.

4. **Don't be afraid to split portions:** If you're eating out and the portion size is too large, it is ok to split the portion. You can ask for a box to take the other half home or share it with a friend.

5. **Be mindful of your portions**: It is important to be mindful of your portion sizes. Ask yourself if you are really hungry or if you are just eating out of habit.

By following these tips, you can measure and control portion sizes to maintain a healthy weight. Remember that portion sizes are important, but they aren't everything. Eating a balanced diet and engaging in regular physical activity are also important for achieving and maintaining a healthy weight.

What Are Healthy Portions: Create Your Plate

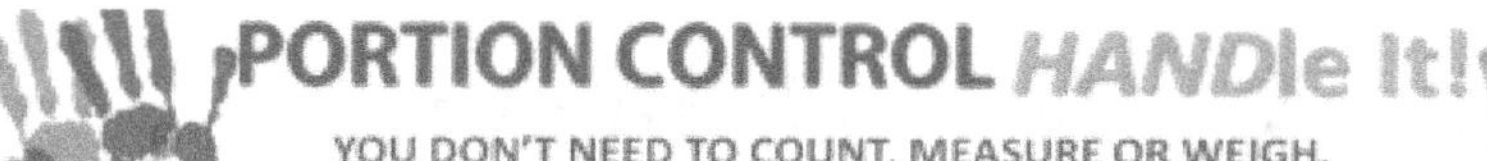

1 PALM = 3 OUNCES
PROTEIN
Meat, Fish, Eggs, Turkey And Chicken

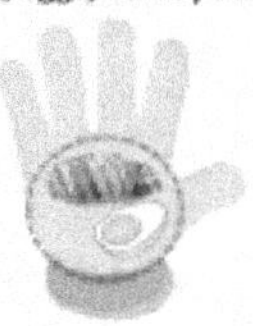

1 WHOLE FIST = 1 CUP
VEGETABLES

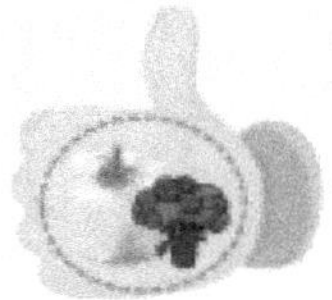

1 CLENCHED FIST = ½ CUP
SIMPLE AND COMPEX CARBOHYDRATES
Grains, Starches, Beans and Fruits

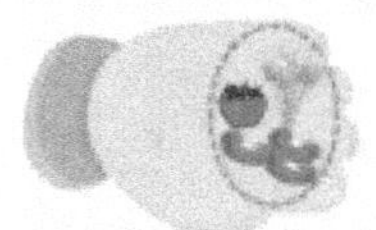

1 THUMB = 1 TABLESPOON
HEALTHY FATS
Oils, Butter, Nuts, Nut Butters, Avocado And Seeds

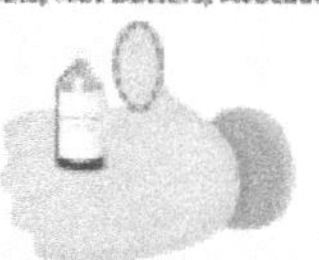

THE HEALTHY PLATE
EAT EVERY 3 HOURS TO KEEP BLOOD SUGARS STABLE

MEN

WOMEN

1 ½ to 2 PALMS OF PROTEIN
Depending On Activity Level
And Muscle Building Activity

1 PALM OF PROTEIN

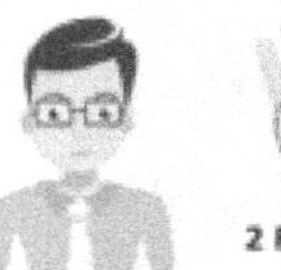
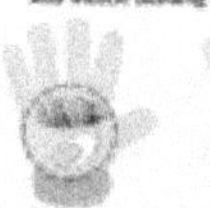
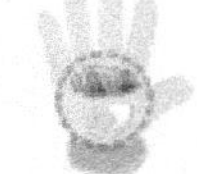

2 FISTS OF VEGETABLES

1 FIST OF VEGETABLES

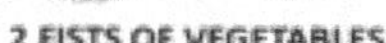
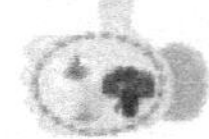

2 CLENCHED FISTS OF CARBS

1 CLENCHED FIST OF CARBS

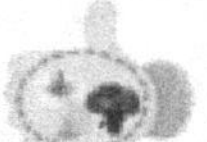
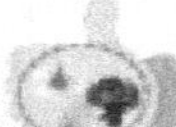
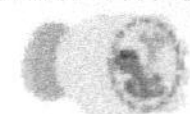

1 THUMB OF FAT

1 THUMB OF FAT

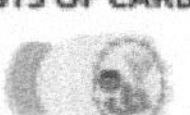
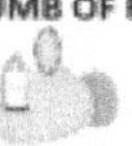

DRINK 4 - 6 QUARTS
OF WATER DAILY

DRINK 2 - 4 QUARTS
OF WATER DAILY

FREE FOODS

HERBS AND ALL SPICES
Garlic
Cilantro
Parsley

FRESH LEAFY GREENS
All Varieties Of Lettuce
Kale
Spinach

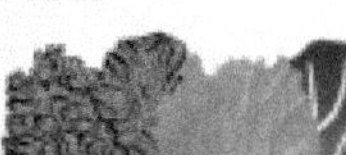
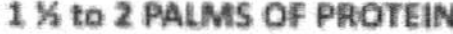

Eat in Moderation

You have heard the saying that everything is good in moderation and it is never more-true than when it comes to food.

Lifestyle change means you can make choices, you are empowered, and you are not deprived.

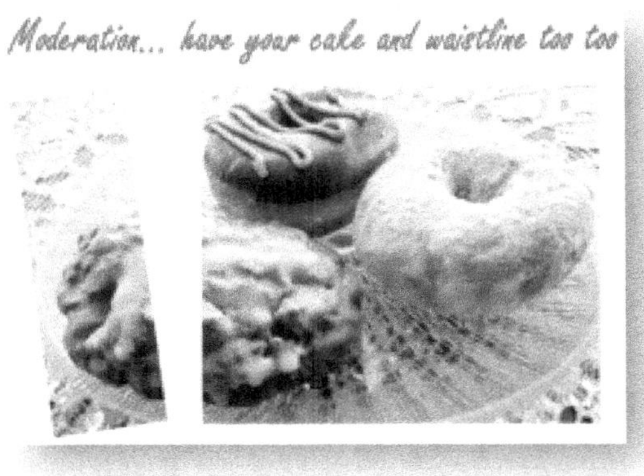

In order to learn moderation, you must learn self-control. Through practicing portion control, you will learn how to use this to your advantage.

For instance, if you are going from drinking six soft drinks a day to replacing three of those with water, you are on the right track. Even though that may still be over the daily limit, you are acting on moderation.

When you are ready to go deeper, you can start dropping more. One soft drink a day is much better in contrast to six.

Moderation means:

✓ Two bites of a donut instead of 3 donuts
✓ 2 bites of cake instead of 1 or 2 slices
✓ A cookie on occasion instead of 6 every day
✓ 1 slice of pizza a week, instead of 3 slices in one sitting
✓ ½ cup of ice cream on game day versus 1/2 a tub every weekend
✓ ¼ cup of mashed potatoes with your dinner, instead of 1 or more cups
✓ ½ a biscuit instead of 3 with dinner

Remember, you are on a path to weight management and a lifestyle change, not a crash diet. It does not have to nor should it happen in a day.

Your Relationship with Food: Eating to Live Versus Living to Eat

In order to be successful throughout this weight management journey, you must change your mindset, and this may require that you improve your relationship with food.

10 Signs of An Unhealthy Relationship with Food

- You think about food all the time
- You punish yourself for breaking your food rules
- You deny yourself the foods you crave
- You have no self-control over food
- You cut out entire food groups
- Your emotions control your eating habits
- You eat the same foods all the time
- You prefer to eat alone
- You are controlled by food rules
- You suffer from food related guilt

Living To Eat

You wake up in the morning and instantly reach for your coffee. Next, you find yourself driving through the nearest fast food lane to grab a breakfast sandwich and another cup of coffee.

Once you get to work, someone brought in cake for another employee's retirement. You tell yourself you have to have a piece because it is there. You find yourself totally ignoring what your body truly needs and discarding it for what your mind wants is "living to eat."

Another example is the person who is hungry, but holds off eating until their favorite television show starts so eating becomes an "event" versus the person who eats when they are hungry period.

Eating to appease emotions, looking forward to eating as if it is an "occasion," feeling high after eating, and craving sweets or fatty foods when stressed out or just because they need to be stimulated are all examples of living to eat.

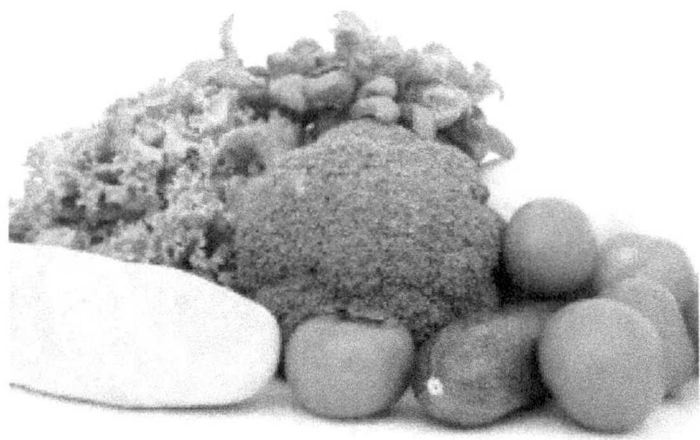

People who "live to eat" often have a negative relationship with food. They tend to over eat their favorites, and even when they are stuffed, they keep eating because the food tastes so good or because it is there. They look forward to meals because they make them happy and they associate eating with happiness.

Many in this predicament do not understand or practice moderation, and they feel guilt and shame associated with what they eat and their eating habits.

Eating To Live

On the other side of the spectrum, is the person who eats to satisfy hunger. They do not have out of control cravings, they eat to satisfaction and not to the point where they are stuffed and cannot breathe.

Food does not control them, they control food. They can choose what they eat and how often. They may indulge occasionally, but they do not feel guilty over what they eat, or the foods they want to eat.

They view and treat food as a necessary part of survival, and recognize that while food can be pleasurable and enjoyable, it is not something required to make them happy. They have a positive relationship with food. All this describes, "eating to live."

Can you see the contrast?

By making healthy choices in our daily lives, we can nourish our bodies the correct way instead of abusing them. Eating to live states that you are giving your body what it needs to function and to remain functional.

You are in tune with your body and you listen to what it needs. Eating healthy means, you must prioritize your well-being. You cannot make damaging excuses and expect to see results. It is important to realize that food is not a friend or a way of life. Food is nourishment to our bodies for health and overall energy.

Food aids us in our daily processes and our bodily functions. Living to eat is dangerous to your health and your self-esteem.

Something as simple as being guided by appetite is often a challenge for those who have a dysfunctional relationship with food.

Powerlessness is often at the core of these issues. Surely, you know someone who decides they want to live a healthier lifestyle; they make the decision, and then follow through. It is not a question of a struggle for them, they just do it.

This is somewhat of a challenge for those who have a negative relationship with food, while the decision can be made, the follow through suffers.

The Solution

In order to lose weight and keep it off, we need to have a healthy relationship with food.

Eat less and move more is the formula for weight loss, but for many it is simply not enough because there must be changes in both perspective and behavior towards food.

What are the benefits of forming a healthy relationship with food?

Eating healthy food is essential for physical and mental health. Forming a healthy relationship with food is the key to maintaining a balanced diet and staying fit. It helps us understand our body's needs, differentiate between cravings and genuine hunger, make informed choices, and enjoy eating without guilt.

A healthy relationship with food can help us to better manage stress levels, reduce the risk of developing chronic diseases, ensure our body gets the right nutrients it needs for optimal functioning, and maintain a healthy weight. It also encourages mindful eating habits which can lead to improved overall wellbeing.

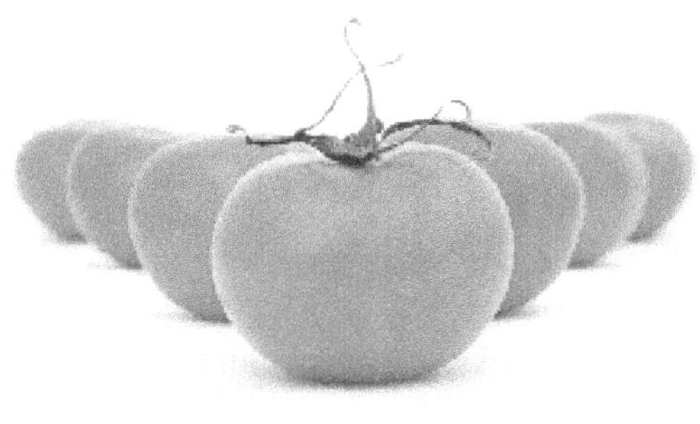

In reality, our mindset needs to change not only in regards to the food choices we make, but also how we relate to that food.

This means learning healthy ways to deal with emotions so not to eat behind them and also changing how we perceive food.

A big part of this process is learning to listen to your body and being able to identify real hunger, versus habitual or dysfunctional eating.

Many people simply cannot identify genuine hunger; this is especially true for emotional eaters who eat behind stress, loneliness, and boredom. There is a better relationship to be had with food. It is time to change this mindset and stop feeling guilty over your choices, get healthy and empowered!

What are the signs that my relationship with food is unhealthy?

Eating is a normal and necessary part of life, but for some people, it can become a source of stress or anxiety. It is important to recognize the signs that your relationship with food has become unhealthy so that you can make changes and regain control.

What strategies can I use to change my relationship with food?

Changing your relationship with food can be a difficult and daunting task but it doesn't have to be. With the right strategies, you can make the transition easier and more enjoyable. From setting realistic goals to experimenting with mindful eating, there are plenty of strategies you can use to create a healthier relationship with food. By understanding your triggers and learning how to manage your emotions, you can start making positive changes that will help you reach your goals.

Simply put, slow down. In other words, take your time and eat.

Allow your body to get the nutrients it needs from whatever you are ingesting. If you feel the urge to grab something quick for lunch for the sake of time, don't do it. Instead, make time for a better meal. Choose healthy and actually sit down to eat. Make time for yourself and your body.

Do Not Eat Emotionally

Emotional eating is a common problem that affects our relationship with food. It can lead to unhealthy eating habits, overeating, and an unhealthy relationship with food. When we emotionally eat, we often turn to comfort foods that are high in sugar and fat, which can lead to weight gain and health problems. Additionally, emotional eating can cause us to ignore our body's signals of hunger and fullness, making it difficult for us to maintain a healthy weight. By understanding the causes of emotional eating and learning healthy coping strategies, we can create a healthier relationship with food.

Minimize Stress

Stress can have a profound impact on our relationship with food. It can lead to unhealthy eating habits, such as overeating or undereating, and can even cause us to turn to food as a source of comfort. Stress can also interfere with our ability to make healthy food choices and can lead us to reach for unhealthy foods as a way of coping. Understanding how stress affects our relationship with food is essential in order to develop healthier eating habits and maintain a balanced diet.

Eat with your body

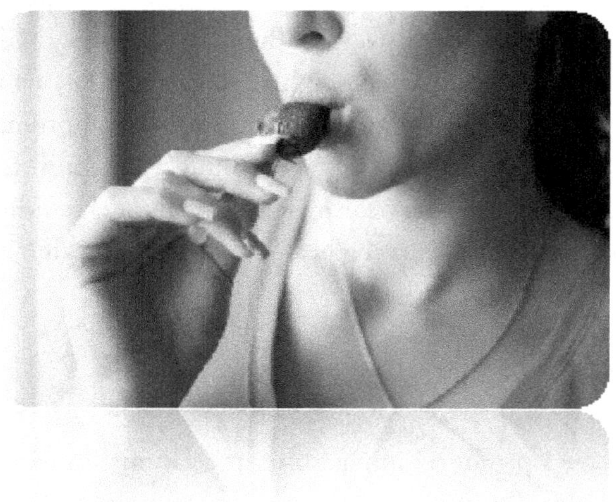

You must start listening to your body, instead of your mind. Our minds can play tricks on us and will make us think we want what we really don't.

Sure, the cake tastes good and we really think we want it. However, does our body need it?

Practice makes perfect with this and as you learn, you will understand what your body is telling you. Think about what will benefit your health instead of what will benefit your impulses.

Instead of trying to satisfy your impulses, learn to satisfy your body's needs.

Yoga can be very helpful in this regard, as it teaches mindfulness and allows practitioners to become much more aware of their body and its needs, including identifying true hunger.

What steps can I take to create a positive attitude towards food?

Creating a positive attitude towards food is an important part of maintaining a healthy lifestyle. It can be difficult to stay motivated and make healthy choices when faced with unhealthy options. However, there are some simple steps you can take to help create a positive attitude towards food. These include setting realistic goals, developing mindful eating habits, and understanding the importance of nutrition. By taking these steps, you will be able to create an attitude that encourages healthy eating and overall wellbeing.

How can I make healthier food choices on a daily basis?

Eating healthy doesn't have to be a chore. With the right knowledge and strategies, you can make healthy food choices every day. From understanding which foods are good for you to learning how to plan meals in advance, making healthier food choices is achievable with a few simple steps. By understanding the nutritional value of different foods and creating an eating plan that works for your lifestyle, you can make healthier food choices on a daily basis and lead a healthier life.

Professional Help

Eating healthy is essential for a healthy lifestyle and overall wellbeing. But it can be difficult to know what foods are best for you and how to make sure you're getting all the nutrients your body needs.

Professional help can be invaluable in this regard, as they can provide advice on how to eat healthily, create meal plans tailored to your individual needs, and offer support when needed.

With professional help, you will have the knowledge and guidance necessary to make informed decisions about what you put in your body. Eating healthy doesn't have to be complicated or boring - it is all about finding the right balance of nutritious foods that work for you.

Weight Control – The Ultimate Goal

Being overweight can have dire consequences in the long run. It is therefore important that a healthy weight be maintained once it is achieved. Maintaining a healthy weight translates to maintaining a healthy lifestyle. However, when weight is not controlled properly, there can be serious consequences for the individual's physical and mental health.

The most obvious consequence of poor weight control is an increased risk of obesity.

Obesity is a serious medical condition that can lead to a range of health problems, such as heart disease, stroke, type 2 diabetes, joint pain, and even some forms of cancer. In addition, obese individuals are more likely to suffer from depression, social isolation, and poor self-esteem.

The rate of obesity in the United States is alarming. More than two-thirds of adults and one-third of children are overweight or obese. This is a serious public health crisis because obesity can increase the risk of many health problems.

Obesity is a complex problem with many causes. It is important to understand the factors involved in order to address the issue. Genetics, lifestyle, and environment all play a role. Genetics may predispose a person to obesity, but lifestyle and environment can be modified to prevent it.

One of the most important lifestyle factors is diet. Incorporating more fresh fruits and vegetables, whole grains, and lean proteins into the diet can help to maintain a healthy weight. Limiting processed and sugary foods can also help. Being physically active is also an important part of an obesity prevention strategy. Aiming for at least 150 minutes of moderate to vigorous activity per week can help to reduce the risk of obesity.

In addition to lifestyle changes, the environment can be modified to promote healthy behaviors. This includes increasing access to nutritious foods, providing safe places to be physically active, and limiting access to unhealthy foods.

The obesity epidemic is a serious public health issue with far-reaching consequences. It is important to understand the causes and take steps to address them. Incorporating healthy eating and physical activity into daily life, as well as making changes to the environment, can help to reduce the risk of obesity and its associated health problems.

Another consequence of poor weight control is an increased risk of developing eating disorders.

Eating disorders are mental illnesses that can have serious physical, psychological, and social effects. These disorders can include anorexia nervosa, bulimia nervosa, and binge eating disorder. Eating disorders can lead to severe nutritional deficiencies and can even be fatal if left untreated.

Poor weight control can also have a negative impact on an individual's quality of life.

People who are overweight or obese may experience difficulties with physical activities, such as running or playing sports. They may also experience physical and emotional pain, a decrease in self-confidence and self-esteem, social isolation, a decreased risk of self-confidence, and a greater risk for developing other chronic health conditions.

Poor weight control can increase the risk of developing certain types of cancer.

Research has shown that being overweight or obese increases the risk of developing certain types of cancers, such as breast, colon, and endometrial cancer.

It is important to maintain a healthy weight in order to avoid the serious consequences associated with poor weight control. Eating a balanced diet and engaging in regular physical activity can help individuals achieve and maintain a healthy weight.

Individuals who are concerned about their weight should also talk to their healthcare provider, who can provide guidance and support.

Weight Control and Blood Sugar

It is also important to understand the way your body's blood sugar works. When you have excess glucose in the blood stream that is 5 grams or more and you consume more carbohydrates such as sugars and starches (potatoes, rice or bread) than what the body immediately needs it produces insulin, which is either it is used immediately for energy, or if there is too much of it is converted to glycogen by the liver and stored as fat.

Your blood sugar must stay regulated to properly aid in healthy weight management

In order to regulate blood sugars it is important to eat every three hours.

Think about how you eat when you are famished? Typically, when people are starved they eat much more food in one sitting than they would otherwise.

When you eat two or 3 big meals a day you tend to go for six to eight hours without food where your blood sugar drops significantly, and then once you do eat you will eat more than a small portion of food and your blood sugar will spike. These spikes cause excess insulin in the blood, which makes the body store fat more easily.

Eating a small meal every 3 hours means

✓ You will never feel starved

✓ You will maintain balanced blood sugar levels

✓ You will avoid overeating and gorging as a result of feeling famished

✓ You will boost your metabolism and turn your body into a fat burning machine

The idea behind eating healthy and keeping weight off for the long-term is not to starve

Remember that starvation is one of the main reasons no one can stick with fad diets on a permanent basis.

Exercise

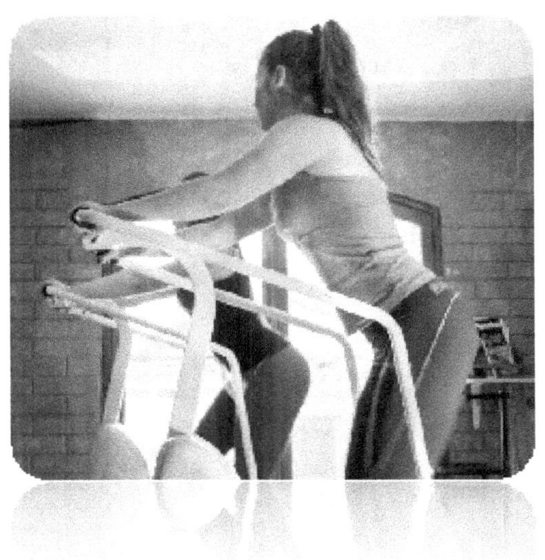

In addition to healthy eating, you should exercise. The Centers for Disease Control advises that engaging in moderate intensive activity for 60 to 90 minutes each week means you are much more likely to keep the weight off over the long term.

You do not have to run 4K marathons. If you can manage 15 to 30 minutes of healthy cardio such as walking or cycling, you are doing better than most.

Exercising may be difficult at first while your body is transitioning from unhealthy to healthy. However, as your body adapts, so will you. Exercise will become less difficult and you will find yourself improving.

The Mayo Clinic states that there are several benefits to exercise including:

✓ Expends energy (calories out)

✓ Allows you to eat more
✓ Reducing risks for heart disease and other chronic conditions
✓ Improved sleep
✓ Supports permanent weight loss
✓ Lowers risk for chronic disease
✓ Boosts energy
✓ Boost brain health
✓ Promotes a positive mood

Empower Yourself with Choices

Making choices about food can be an empowering experience. One of the greatest things about a new lifestyle, versus being "on a diet" is that you have choices. Unlike drastic and fad diets, you are not deprived and you are not restricted.

You get to make choices about both food and exercise, which can empower you. A new lifestyle allows you to make **mindful decisions** about what you eat, how you eat and exercise.

It can help you take control of your health, your diet, and your wellbeing. You can make informed decisions about which foods to incorporate into your daily meals and snacks that will help you reach your personal health and wellness goals.

Taking the time to research the best nutrition for you and your lifestyle can be incredibly rewarding. By looking into the various components of nutrition, from macronutrients such as protein and carbohydrates to micronutrients like vitamins and minerals, you can ensure that you are getting the most out of your meals.

Additionally, understanding the different types of fats and how they affect your body can help you make more informed decisions about the types of fats you eat.

Taking into account your individual dietary needs and preferences can help you create an eating plan that works for you.

An important part of making food choices that work for you is taking into account your values, preferences, and lifestyle.

Incorporating mindful eating practices can also help you make more mindful and informed food choice decisions.

Mindful eating involves being aware of the physical and mental signals your body sends when you are hungry and full and responding with intentional choices that adhere to your needs and values.

All in all, making conscious choices about food can be an empowering experience that will help you reach your personal health and wellness goals and improve your overall wellbeing.

Recap: Permanent Weight Loss Formula Steps

As you can see, the permanent weight loss formula is not another diet. This is a complete lifestyle change that empowers you with choices and resets old habits to new and healthier ones.

Each habit takes you closer to your weight loss goals, and once
those habits are set, you can keep the weight off, and NEVER diet again!

RECAP OF THE PERMANENT WEIGHT LOSS FORMULA:

Make Habit Changes Your Goal Instead of Weight Loss

Calories In - Calories Out

Balanced Eating Plan

Portion Control

Eat Every 3 Hours to Stabilize Blood Sugars

Eat in Moderation

Exercise (Calories Out)

These are the key aspects of healthy and permanent weight loss. The key is to not starve and to stay active. Your body must have all food groups to remain healthy. Portion control is important for calorie control. Moderation is important for those not so healthy treats.

Your blood sugar must be stabilized in order for your body to react properly. Exercise is needed to seal the deal between healthy weight loss and your actions. Improving your relationship with food will allow you to achieve these steps, and provide you with the self-control and perception needed to succeed.

Are There Any Lifestyle Change Commercial Diets?

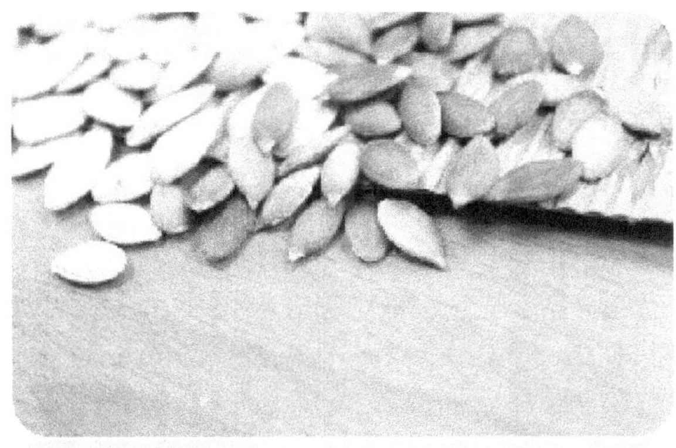

Lifestyle change diets are an effective way to lose weight in a healthy and sustainable way. It is all about making healthy choices that are good for your body and mind. When you change your lifestyle for the better, you will be able to enjoy the benefits of a healthier and happier life.

The first step to making a lifestyle change is to make a commitment to yourself. Make a commitment to eating healthier foods, exercising regularly, managing stress and getting enough sleep.

Eating healthy foods is key to losing weight and keeping it off. Focus on eating whole, unprocessed foods such as fruits, vegetables, whole grains, lean proteins, and healthy fats. Limit foods that are high in added sugars and unhealthy fats. Exercise regularly to help boost your metabolism and burn calories.

Aim for 30 minutes of moderate physical activity most days of the week. Incorporate strength training exercises to help build muscle, which helps to burn more calories. Managing stress is also important for weight loss and overall health.

Take time each day to relax and decompress. Get enough sleep to help your body recover after a hard day.

A Lifestyle change diet is an excellent way to achieve sustainable weight loss and improved health. Making lifestyle changes can help you reach your weight loss goals, while also improving your mental and physical wellbeing.

You may be thinking, "Sure, I can change my lifestyle, but I think I might need some help getting there." There are actual lifestyle change diets that do exist, but only a few. These diets focus on changing your actual eating habits to promote permanent weight loss instead of losing weight quickly with a temporary diet. One of these lifestyle change diets is Weight Watchers™.

What is Weight Watchers?

Weight Watchers is not a diet, but a lifestyle change plan. They take into account each body type and customize a plan just for you.

Weight Watchers will support and teach you to make better food choices.

You can choose to attend weekly meetings or online or a combination of both depending on your changing needs.

What makes Weight Watchers a real lifestyle change diet?

- **Teaches you to eat correctly** - Weight Watchers does not make you drop everything you enjoy. Instead, they show you how to eat correctly by using their SmartPoints system and by eating from all food groups.

There are absolutely no foods that are off limits on this program, instead members get to choose what they want based on a point system as long as they do not go over their daily point limit.

This allows members to actually make changes through choices. Since the higher point foods are typically sweets and more unhealthy items, choosing them means eating less food overall during that day, versus choosing something more healthy that's worth less points.

There is no deprivation, just choices, and through this process, members are empowered and learn to make healthier choices.

- **Exercise is included** – This program smartly includes exercise, where active people get a higher point allowance allowing them to eat more.

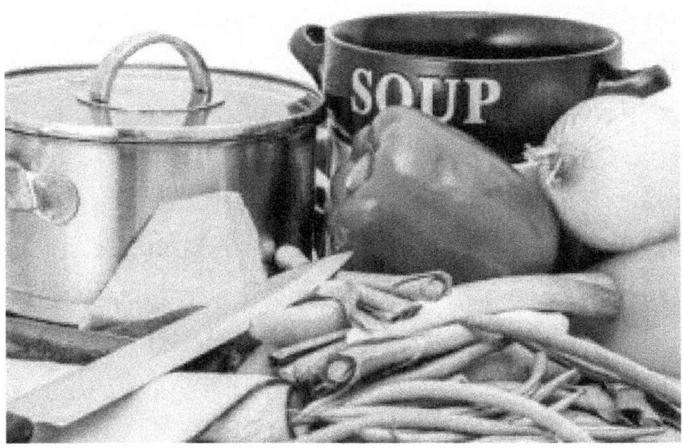

- **Teaches portion control** - With Weight Watchers' point system, portions determine points assigned. This teaches you to eat smaller portions of the foods you love instead of all. Since learning moderation is key in making healthy habit changes, this allows members to realize that they can have a cookie, and they do not need to feel deprived or guilty about losing weight. Portion control also changes attitudes towards eating smaller portions while realizing that satisfaction is possible while doing so.

- **Provides support** - You are not alone in this system. There are plenty of ways to reach out and gain support. Weight Watchers has weekly weigh-ins and meetings where you can go and voice you frustrations and thoughts and reach out to others. There is also an online community where you can share and meet others going through the program. There are plenty of helpful resources available to you online as well.
- **Follow on your own** - Weight Watchers happens at your own pace. You are not trying to lose a ton of weight all at once. Instead, you are changing your life. This program is not difficult to learn and is not difficult to keep up with. You can follow along on your own, if you wish, and take it one day at a time. This creates a way for you to slowly add these things into your life without feeling overwhelmed.

Weight Watchers is a lifestyle change program that will allow to eat healthier and engage you in the process of making healthy choices.

Keep in mind that you can lose weight and keep it off on your own by following the Weight Loss Formula discussed, and you do not have to pay for Weight Watchers, but it is something to consider for those who would like a more structured approach.

Although Weight Watchers is a very good program to use for weight loss, there are alternatives available.

Some of these alternative programs also exist in the form of apps that can be used to track calories, exercise and other physical activity. These are all designed to assist you in the weight loss process.

A quick Internet search will provide more information based on the list below:

- iTrackbites
- Lose It
- Mayo Clinic Diet
- MyFitnesspal
- Lifesum
- Noom

Final Thoughts

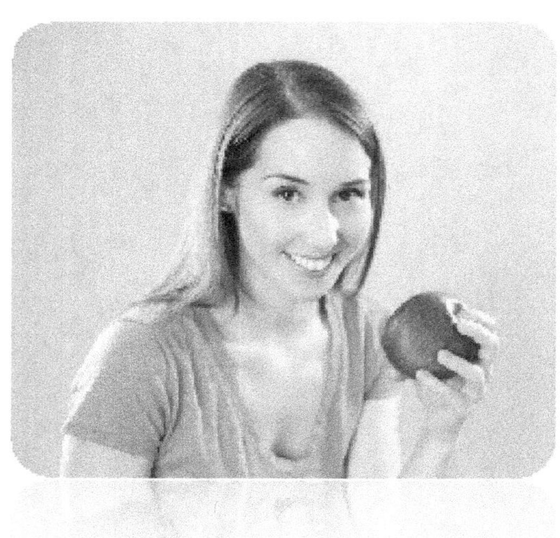

We have discussed many things including how to change your mindset and how to reclaim your relationship with food.

However, the most important takeaway is for you to understand the importance of valuing yourself and your health.

Above anything else, you should do what makes you healthier and your body stronger. Rome wasn't built in a day and neither are you.

Take time to make a plan and stick to it, when you make mistakes learn from them and move on.

Eating should not make you feel guilty. Instead, it should empower you. Food was created to nourish our bodies, not control them.

Start out small and make changes consistently.

Make Habit Changes Your Goal and Not Weight Loss

Don't worry if the weight loss is slow, this is actually a much healthier way to lose and more sustainable than quick drastic losses.

The long-term benefits of weight management outweigh the short-term benefits of crash dieting. It is better for your health.

You are worth more than living deprived,
so ditch the diet mindset, and start living!

Further Reading

68

Cleveland Clinic. (2020, August 4). Fad diets.
    https://my.clevelandclinic.org/health/articles/9476-fad-diets

Shmerling, R. H. (2023, April 1). Mastering portion control for effective weight loss.
    https://chgeharvard.org/mastering-portion-control-for-effective-weight-loss/

Thorpe, M. (2017, May 29). 10 solid reasons why Yo-Yo dieting is bad for you.
    https://www.healthline.com/nutrition/yo-yo-dieting
    | Page